Chapter 1: Understanding Vascular Dementia

Definition and Overview

Vascular dementia is a form of cognitive decline caused by reduced blood flow to the brain, often resulting from strokes or other conditions that damage blood vessels. This type of dementia is characterized by a decline in thinking skills, memory, and the ability to perform everyday activities. Understanding vascular dementia is crucial for families and patients as early detection can significantly influence the management and progression of the disease. Symptoms may vary widely among individuals but often include difficulties with problem-solving, confusion, and changes in mood and behavior.

The onset of vascular dementia typically follows a stepwise pattern, with symptoms worsening after each vascular event, such as a stroke. This distinguishes it from other forms of dementia, like Alzheimer's disease, which tends to show a gradual decline. Recognizing the early signs and symptoms is essential for families to seek timely medical intervention. Early diagnosis can lead to better management strategies that can help maintain cognitive function and quality of life for as long as possible.

Effective diagnosis of vascular dementia involves a thorough evaluation that includes medical history, neurological examinations, cognitive testing, and brain imaging techniques such as MRI or CT scans. These assessments help in identifying the extent of vascular damage and ruling out other potential causes of cognitive decline. Families should be prepared to discuss any changes they have observed in their loved one's behavior or cognitive abilities with healthcare providers, as this information is vital for an accurate diagnosis.

Once diagnosed, a comprehensive approach to treatment is often necessary. This may include pharmacological interventions aimed at managing symptoms and addressing underlying vascular health issues. Additionally, cognitive rehabilitation techniques can support patients in maintaining cognitive function. Nutrition and lifestyle interventions play a critical role in managing vascular dementia, highlighting the importance of a heart-healthy diet and regular physical activity to promote overall vascular health.

Support for caregivers is equally important in managing vascular dementia. Caregivers often face emotional and physical challenges, and access to community resources can provide essential assistance. Emphasizing the need for support networks can empower families to navigate the complexities of care and improve the quality of life for both patients and caregivers. Understanding the broad landscape of vascular dementia, including its implications for daily living and the importance of ethical considerations in care, is vital for families as they embark on this journey.

Causes and Risk Factors

Vascular dementia is primarily caused by reduced blood flow to the brain, which leads to the death of brain cells. This reduction in blood flow can result from various vascular conditions, including strokes, small vessel disease, and other cardiovascular issues. A stroke, whether it is ischemic (caused by a blocked blood vessel) or hemorrhagic (caused by bleeding), can create immediate damage to brain tissue, leading to sudden cognitive changes. However, vascular dementia can also develop over time as a result of multiple smaller strokes or chronic conditions affecting blood circulation, such as high blood pressure and diabetes. Understanding these underlying causes is crucial for families and patients in recognizing early signs and symptoms.

Several risk factors contribute to the likelihood of developing vascular dementia. Age is a significant factor, with individuals over the age of 65 being at higher risk. Additionally, lifestyle choices, such as smoking, excessive alcohol consumption, and physical inactivity, can increase the risk. Chronic health conditions, including hypertension, diabetes, and high cholesterol, play a pivotal role in vascular health. Genetic predispositions and family history of dementia can also elevate risk levels. By identifying these risk factors, families can take proactive measures to modify lifestyle choices and manage health conditions that can contribute to cognitive decline.

The interplay between vascular health and cognitive function cannot be overstated. Conditions that affect the heart and blood vessels, such as atherosclerosis (the buildup of fatty deposits in arteries), directly impact blood flow to the brain. Maintaining cardiovascular health through regular exercise, a balanced diet, and routine medical check-ups can be instrumental in reducing the risk of vascular dementia. Research indicates that interventions focusing on vascular health not only support brain function but can also mitigate the progression of cognitive decline in individuals already diagnosed with vascular dementia.

Nutrition and lifestyle interventions are essential components of managing risk factors and promoting overall brain health. A diet rich in fruits, vegetables, whole grains, and lean proteins can support vascular function and cognitive health. The Mediterranean diet, for instance, has been associated with lower risks of cognitive decline. Regular physical activity, such as walking or swimming, enhances blood circulation and can help maintain cognitive function. Additionally, addressing mental health through stress-reduction techniques and social engagement can also play a significant role in preventing vascular dementia.

Finally, awareness of the ethical considerations in managing vascular dementia is crucial for families and caregivers. As cognitive function declines, patients may face challenges in making decisions about their care and lifestyle. Open communication, advance care planning, and involving patients in decision-making processes are essential for respecting their autonomy and wishes. Families should also be aware of community resources and support networks available for individuals living with vascular dementia, which can provide valuable assistance and guidance in navigating the complexities of the condition.

Symptoms and Stages

Symptoms of vascular dementia can vary significantly among individuals, but there are common signs that families and patients should be aware of. Early symptoms often include confusion, difficulty concentrating, and trouble with organization and planning. Patients may experience challenges in their ability to follow conversations or keep track of their thoughts. As vascular dementia progresses, changes in mood and behavior may also manifest, leading to increased irritability, anxiety, or depression. Recognizing these early symptoms is crucial for timely intervention and management.

The progression of vascular dementia can be categorized into stages, each characterized by distinct symptoms and challenges. In the early stage, cognitive impairment may be subtle, often mistaken for normal aging. As the disease advances to the middle stage, individuals may face greater difficulties with daily tasks, such as managing finances or maintaining personal hygiene. At this point, families may notice a more pronounced decline in memory and an increase in confusion. Understanding these stages can help families prepare for the changes that lie ahead and foster a supportive environment for the affected individual.

As vascular dementia progresses to the later stages, patients may become increasingly dependent on caregivers for assistance with daily activities. Communication may deteriorate, making it challenging for patients to express their needs or engage in conversations. Physical symptoms may also present, such as difficulty walking or an increased risk of falls. Caregivers play a vital role in providing support and ensuring safety, and it is essential for families to recognize the strain that these changes can place on both the patient and the caregiver.

Effective management of vascular dementia requires a comprehensive approach that includes cognitive rehabilitation techniques, nutrition, and lifestyle interventions. Engaging patients in activities that stimulate cognitive function, such as puzzles or memory games, can be beneficial. Likewise, a balanced diet rich in fruits, vegetables, and omega-3 fatty acids may support vascular health and cognitive function. Families should also promote physical activity and social engagement, as these elements can significantly impact overall well-being and quality of life for individuals living with vascular dementia.

Support for families and caregivers is critical in navigating the complexities of vascular dementia. Various resources are available, including support groups and educational programs that can provide valuable information and emotional support. Understanding the ethical considerations in managing care and making decisions for a loved one can also be challenging. By accessing community resources and fostering open communication, families can create a supportive network that not only aids in the care of the affected individual but also addresses the emotional and psychological needs of the caregiver.

Chapter 2: Early Detection and Diagnosis

Importance of Early Detection

Early detection of vascular dementia is crucial for both patients and their families, as it allows for timely interventions that can significantly improve the quality of life. Recognizing the early signs of cognitive decline can lead to prompt medical evaluations, which are essential for accurate diagnosis and management. This proactive approach not only helps in understanding the condition but also enables families to make informed decisions regarding care and treatment. The earlier the diagnosis, the more effective the strategies can be in mitigating symptoms and maintaining cognitive function.

Identifying vascular dementia in its initial stages can also open the door to various rehabilitation techniques tailored to the specific needs of the patient. Cognitive rehabilitation strategies, for instance, are most effective when implemented early. Patients may benefit from personalized interventions designed to enhance cognitive skills, improve memory, and foster independence. Family members play a crucial role in this process, as engagement and support from loved ones can accelerate recovery and adaptation to changes in cognitive function.

Nutrition and lifestyle interventions are other critical aspects of managing vascular dementia that are best initiated early. A balanced diet rich in nutrients that support brain health, coupled with regular physical activity, can help in slowing the progression of the disease. Families can work together to create an environment that encourages healthy eating habits and active living. Educating family members on the significance of vascular health is vital; they can help ensure that patients adhere to lifestyle changes that may minimize further vascular deterioration.

Moreover, early detection provides families with the opportunity to explore pharmacological treatments that can stabilize or improve symptoms. Medications tailored to address vascular dementia can be more effective when started early in the disease process. Families should be informed about available treatments and should engage in discussions with healthcare providers about the best options for their loved ones. This collaborative approach can lead to improved outcomes and help manage the complexities associated with the condition.

Finally, the impact of vascular dementia on daily living activities can be substantial, making it essential for families to understand the importance of early detection. Recognizing changes in behavior or cognitive function allows families to adapt their caregiving strategies accordingly. Accessing community resources and support networks is also facilitated by an early diagnosis, as families can connect with organizations that provide valuable information and assistance. In conclusion, early detection not only enhances the management of vascular dementia but also empowers families to navigate the challenges that come with the condition, ensuring a better quality of life for both patients and caregivers.

Diagnostic Tools and Assessments

Diagnostic tools and assessments play a crucial role in identifying vascular dementia at an early stage. These assessments typically begin with a thorough medical history and a comprehensive evaluation of cognitive function. Family members often provide valuable insights into the patient's daily life and any noticeable changes in behavior, memory, or reasoning. This information helps healthcare professionals determine the most appropriate diagnostic path. A combination of clinical interviews, standardized tests, and physical exams allows for a detailed understanding of the individual's cognitive abilities and overall health.

Neuropsychological testing is one of the most effective methods for assessing cognitive function in patients suspected of having vascular dementia. These tests evaluate various cognitive domains, including memory, attention, language, and executive function. The results can help differentiate vascular dementia from other types of dementia, such as Alzheimer's disease, as they provide a clearer picture of how vascular issues are affecting cognitive abilities. Family members may be involved in these assessments, as their observations can highlight specific cognitive challenges faced by their loved ones.

Imaging technologies, such as magnetic resonance imaging (MRI) and computed tomography (CT) scans, are essential diagnostic tools in the evaluation of vascular dementia. These imaging techniques help visualize the brain's structure and identify any vascular damage, such as lesions or strokes. The presence of these abnormalities can correlate with cognitive decline, reinforcing the diagnosis of vascular dementia. Family members should understand the significance of these imaging results, as they provide critical information about the underlying causes of cognitive impairment.

In addition to cognitive assessments and imaging, laboratory tests are often conducted to rule out other medical conditions that may mimic or contribute to cognitive decline. Blood tests can check for vitamin deficiencies, thyroid function, and other metabolic issues that could affect brain health. Understanding the full medical context of a patient's cognitive difficulties is vital for accurate diagnosis and effective intervention. Families are encouraged to participate actively in discussions about laboratory findings, as this knowledge can empower them to make informed decisions regarding their loved one's care.

Finally, ongoing monitoring and reassessment are vital components of managing vascular dementia. As the condition progresses, it is essential to regularly evaluate cognitive function and adjust care strategies accordingly. This may involve changes in medications, lifestyle interventions, or rehabilitation techniques tailored to the patient's evolving needs. Families should be proactive in seeking updates from healthcare providers and engaging in discussions about the best approaches to support their loved ones. By understanding the diagnostic tools and assessments available, families can play an active role in the early detection and management of vascular dementia, ultimately enhancing the quality of life for both patients and caregivers.

Working with Healthcare Professionals

Working with healthcare professionals is a crucial aspect of navigating vascular dementia for both patients and their families. Establishing a collaborative relationship with doctors, nurses, and therapists can significantly impact the early detection, diagnosis, and management of vascular dementia. Family members should take an active role in this partnership, ensuring that they communicate openly and effectively with healthcare providers. This involves discussing symptoms, concerns, and any changes observed in the patient's behavior or daily functioning. Recognizing the importance of these interactions can foster a supportive environment that prioritizes the patient's health and well-being.

In the context of early detection and diagnosis, healthcare professionals utilize various assessment tools and diagnostic criteria to evaluate cognitive changes. Families should be vigilant in observing behavioral shifts and cognitive decline, as these insights can aid in prompting timely medical consultations. When visiting a healthcare provider, it is helpful for families to prepare a list of questions and concerns, as well as to provide detailed observations of any changes in the patient's cognitive abilities and daily activities. This proactive approach not only aids in accurate diagnosis but also ensures that the healthcare professional has a comprehensive understanding of the patient's condition.

Once a diagnosis of vascular dementia is established, healthcare professionals play a vital role in creating a comprehensive care plan. This plan may include cognitive rehabilitation techniques aimed at enhancing the patient's cognitive functioning and daily living skills. Families can collaborate with occupational and speech therapists to implement these strategies effectively at home. Understanding the therapeutic interventions available, such as memory exercises and problem-solving activities, empowers families to support their loved ones in maintaining independence and quality of life.

Nutrition and lifestyle interventions are also essential components of managing vascular dementia. Healthcare professionals can provide guidance on dietary modifications, physical activity recommendations, and lifestyle changes that promote vascular health. Families should engage in discussions about the benefits of a heart-healthy diet and regular exercise, as these factors can influence the progression of dementia. By working together with healthcare providers, families can help create an environment that fosters healthier habits, which may contribute positively to the patient's cognitive function and overall health.

Finally, ongoing communication with healthcare professionals is vital for caregiver support. Caregivers often face significant emotional and physical challenges while caring for someone with vascular dementia. Healthcare providers can offer resources, support groups, and counseling services that address caregiver needs. Families should not hesitate to seek assistance, as this can alleviate stress and improve the overall caregiving experience. By fostering a strong support network with healthcare professionals, families can navigate the complexities of vascular dementia more effectively, ensuring better outcomes for both patients and caregivers alike.

Chapter 3: Cognitive Rehabilitation Techniques

Overview of Cognitive Rehabilitation

Cognitive rehabilitation is a structured approach aimed at improving cognitive functions that may be impaired due to vascular dementia. This process is designed to help patients regain or compensate for lost skills, enhancing their ability to manage daily activities and maintain independence. Cognitive rehabilitation typically involves a variety of therapeutic techniques that can be tailored to the individual's specific deficits, focusing on areas such as memory, attention, problem-solving, and executive function. By addressing these cognitive challenges, families can help their loved ones navigate the complexities of vascular dementia and improve their overall quality of life.

The foundation of cognitive rehabilitation lies in understanding the unique cognitive profile of each patient. Assessments conducted by healthcare professionals identify specific areas of difficulty, allowing for the development of personalized rehabilitation plans. These plans may include exercises aimed at improving memory recall, enhancing attention span, or teaching compensatory strategies that help patients cope with cognitive limitations. This individualized approach not only fosters a sense of achievement in patients but also empowers families by providing them with tools to support their loved ones effectively.

Incorporating lifestyle interventions, such as nutrition and physical activity, plays a crucial role in cognitive rehabilitation. A balanced diet rich in antioxidants, omega-3 fatty acids, and other essential nutrients has been shown to positively affect cognitive health. Additionally, engaging in regular physical exercise can improve blood flow to the brain, potentially slowing the progression of vascular dementia. Family members can encourage these healthy habits by participating in meal planning and physical activities together, creating a supportive environment that reinforces the principles of cognitive rehabilitation.

Caregiver support strategies are also essential in the context of cognitive rehabilitation. Family members often face significant emotional and physical demands while caring for a loved one with vascular dementia. Providing caregivers with resources, such as support groups and educational materials, can help them manage stress and enhance their ability to assist the patient. By fostering an open dialogue about the challenges faced, families can work together to develop effective coping mechanisms and ensure that both patients and caregivers feel supported throughout the rehabilitation process.

Research continues to advance our understanding of cognitive rehabilitation strategies in vascular dementia. Emerging studies highlight the effectiveness of various therapeutic techniques, such as cognitive training, mindfulness practices, and technology-assisted interventions. As new findings are integrated into rehabilitation programs, families can remain informed about the latest advancements and best practices in managing vascular dementia. Engaging in discussions with healthcare providers about these developments can empower families to make informed decisions regarding their loved ones' care, ultimately contributing to a more hopeful outlook in the journey through vascular dementia.

Effective Strategies and Exercises

Effective strategies and exercises play a crucial role in managing vascular dementia, particularly in the early stages when intervention can significantly improve quality of life. Families and caregivers can adopt a holistic approach that encompasses cognitive rehabilitation techniques, lifestyle adjustments, and nutritional support. These strategies are not only beneficial for the person living with vascular dementia but also provide essential assistance to caregivers, fostering a supportive environment that promotes mental and physical health.

Cognitive rehabilitation techniques are designed to help patients retain and improve cognitive functions. Simple exercises such as memory games, puzzles, and reading can stimulate brain activity and foster engagement. Incorporating activities that encourage reminiscence, like sharing memories or looking through photo albums, can also be effective. Such exercises not only help maintain cognitive abilities but also strengthen the emotional bond between patients and their families, creating a nurturing atmosphere conducive to mental well-being.

Nutrition and lifestyle interventions are equally important in managing vascular dementia. A diet rich in fruits, vegetables, whole grains, and lean proteins can support vascular health, potentially slowing the progression of dementia. Omega-3 fatty acids, found in fish and nuts, are particularly beneficial for brain health. Additionally, regular physical activity, tailored to the individual's capabilities, can improve circulation and overall health, further reducing the risk of cognitive decline. Family involvement in these lifestyle changes can enhance motivation and adherence, making it a shared journey toward better health.

Caregiver support strategies are vital in ensuring that caregivers do not experience burnout while providing care. Establishing a routine that includes scheduled breaks and self-care activities can help caregivers maintain their mental and physical health. Engaging in support groups can also provide caregivers with valuable resources and emotional support, allowing them to share experiences and coping strategies with others in similar situations. This network can be essential in navigating the challenges that arise with vascular dementia, offering both practical advice and emotional reassurance.

Finally, staying informed about medications and pharmacological treatments is essential for managing vascular dementia effectively. Collaborating with healthcare professionals to find the most appropriate treatment plan can optimize cognitive function and manage behavioral symptoms. Keeping abreast of research advances in vascular dementia can empower families with knowledge about potential new therapies and interventions. This proactive approach not only benefits the individual with vascular dementia but also helps families feel more in control of the situation, fostering a proactive rather than reactive stance in their caregiving journey.

Role of Therapy in Rehabilitation

The role of therapy in the rehabilitation of individuals with vascular dementia is multifaceted, addressing both cognitive and emotional needs. Therapy can help patients regain lost cognitive functions or develop strategies to cope with deficits, enhancing their overall quality of life. Cognitive rehabilitation techniques focus on improving memory, attention, and executive functioning through structured exercises and activities tailored to the individual's capabilities. This personalized approach not only aids in cognitive recovery but also fosters a sense of accomplishment and motivation.

In addition to cognitive rehabilitation, psychological therapy plays a crucial role in supporting emotional well-being. Individuals diagnosed with vascular dementia may experience feelings of frustration, anxiety, or depression as they navigate their changing cognitive landscape. Therapeutic interventions such as counseling and support groups provide a safe space for patients to express their emotions, share experiences, and connect with others facing similar challenges. This social support can significantly alleviate feelings of isolation and promote resilience.

Another key aspect of therapy in rehabilitation is the incorporation of lifestyle interventions. Nutrition and physical activity have been shown to have a profound impact on brain health and cognitive function. Therapists often collaborate with nutritionists to develop meal plans that support vascular health, while also encouraging regular physical activity tailored to the patient's abilities. These lifestyle changes can help mitigate further cognitive decline and improve overall health, reinforcing the importance of a holistic approach to rehabilitation.

Family involvement is essential in the therapeutic process, as caregivers play a pivotal role in the rehabilitation journey. Training and support for caregivers can enhance their ability to assist patients with daily activities and therapeutic exercises. Family therapy sessions can also help improve communication and understanding among family members, fostering a supportive environment that is conducive to rehabilitation. This collaborative approach ensures that patients feel supported both emotionally and physically, which is critical for their progress.

Finally, ongoing research into the efficacy of various therapeutic interventions continues to shape the landscape of rehabilitation for vascular dementia. Emerging studies highlight the importance of individualized therapy plans that adapt to the patient's evolving needs. By staying informed about the latest advancements in therapy and rehabilitation techniques, families can advocate for the best possible care for their loved ones. Engaging with community resources and support networks can further enhance the therapeutic experience, ensuring patients and families have access to comprehensive care and support throughout the rehabilitation process.

Chapter 4: Nutrition and Lifestyle Interventions

Dietary Recommendations for Brain Health

Dietary choices play a crucial role in maintaining brain health and can significantly influence the progression of vascular dementia. A well-balanced diet rich in specific nutrients is essential for supporting cognitive function and overall vascular health. Families and patients should focus on incorporating foods that promote brain health, such as fruits, vegetables, whole grains, lean proteins, and healthy fats. These food groups provide essential vitamins, antioxidants, and fatty acids that can help protect the brain from oxidative stress and inflammation, both of which are linked to cognitive decline.

The Mediterranean diet is often highlighted for its benefits in reducing the risk of dementia. This diet emphasizes the consumption of olive oil, fish, nuts, legumes, and a variety of fruits and vegetables. It is low in saturated fats and high in omega-3 fatty acids, which are known to support brain health. Families can consider meal planning that includes these elements, ensuring that meals are not only nutritious but also enjoyable. Engaging in cooking together can foster social interaction and improve mood, which is particularly beneficial for those affected by vascular dementia.

In addition to focusing on what to eat, it is equally important to consider what to limit or avoid. Diets high in refined sugars, saturated fats, and processed foods can contribute to inflammation and vascular problems, which may exacerbate cognitive decline. Families should aim to reduce the intake of sugary snacks, soft drinks, and fast food. Instead, healthy snacks such as nuts, yogurt, and fresh fruits can be substituted, providing necessary nutrients without the harmful effects of processed options.

Hydration is another key aspect of dietary recommendations for brain health. Proper hydration is crucial for maintaining cognitive function, and dehydration can lead to confusion and increased cognitive impairment. Families should encourage regular fluid intake throughout the day, focusing on water and other hydrating beverages. Herbal teas and broths can also be excellent options. Monitoring fluid intake becomes especially important for caregivers, as individuals with vascular dementia may have difficulty recognizing their thirst.

Finally, it is essential to approach dietary changes with consideration for individual preferences and cultural practices. Involving patients in the planning and preparation of meals can create a sense of autonomy and enjoyment around food. Caregivers should take the time to learn about the food preferences of their loved ones and try to incorporate familiar dishes that align with healthy dietary guidelines. This personalized approach not only enhances nutritional intake but also promotes emotional well-being, which is vital for those living with vascular dementia.

Physical Activity and Its Benefits

Physical activity plays a crucial role in maintaining overall health and well-being, particularly for individuals at risk of or living with vascular dementia. Engaging in regular physical activity helps improve cardiovascular health, which is directly linked to brain health. The brain relies on a robust blood supply to function optimally, and activities that promote cardiovascular fitness, such as walking, swimming, or cycling, can enhance blood flow to the brain. This increased circulation can support cognitive function, potentially delaying the onset or progression of vascular dementia symptoms.

Moreover, physical activity has been shown to have positive effects on mood and mental health. Individuals with vascular dementia often experience feelings of depression or anxiety, which can exacerbate cognitive decline. Exercise releases endorphins, the body's natural mood lifters, and can create a sense of accomplishment and improved self-esteem. For caregivers and family members, encouraging a loved one to engage in physical activity can also foster a supportive environment, reducing feelings of isolation and enhancing social interactions, which are essential for emotional well-being.

Incorporating physical activity into daily routines does not have to be overwhelming. Simple adjustments, such as taking short walks, gardening, or participating in light stretching exercises, can be beneficial. Family members can play a supportive role by joining in these activities, creating a shared experience that promotes bonding and motivation. Additionally, structured exercise programs designed for older adults can provide a safe and effective way for individuals with vascular dementia to engage in physical activity while ensuring their specific needs are met.

Research indicates that consistent physical activity can also improve functional abilities in patients with vascular dementia. Regular movement can enhance coordination and balance, reducing the risk of falls, which is a common concern for this population. Additionally, physical activity can help maintain independence in daily living activities, allowing individuals to perform tasks such as dressing, eating, and bathing with greater ease. This preservation of functional abilities is crucial for maintaining quality of life and reducing the burden on caregivers.

In conclusion, the benefits of physical activity extend beyond mere physical health; they encompass emotional, cognitive, and functional improvements that are vital for individuals living with vascular dementia. By prioritizing physical activity and integrating it into daily life, families can help mitigate the impacts of vascular dementia, promote overall health, and foster a supportive environment. Encouraging active lifestyles not only benefits the individual with vascular dementia but also strengthens relationships among family members, creating a more positive and hopeful atmosphere for everyone involved.

Mindfulness and Stress Reduction Techniques

Mindfulness and stress reduction techniques can play a significant role in managing the emotional and psychological challenges associated with vascular dementia. The diagnosis of vascular dementia often brings anxiety and uncertainty for both patients and their families. Practicing mindfulness helps individuals focus on the present moment, alleviating feelings of stress and worry about the future. Techniques such as deep breathing, meditation, and guided imagery can serve as effective tools for calming the mind, enhancing emotional resilience, and fostering a sense of control in an otherwise unpredictable situation.

One effective mindfulness technique is deep breathing exercises, which can be easily integrated into daily routines. By encouraging slow, deliberate breaths, individuals can activate their body's relaxation response, reducing physiological symptoms of stress such as elevated heart rate and muscle tension. Families can practice these exercises together, creating a shared experience that not only promotes relaxation but also strengthens emotional bonds. Setting aside even a few minutes daily for this practice can yield significant benefits in managing stress levels for both patients and caregivers.

Meditation is another valuable technique that can be tailored to suit individual preferences and abilities. Simple mindfulness meditation, which involves focusing on the breath or a specific thought, can help clear the mind of distractions and promote a sense of calm. For those who may find traditional meditation challenging, alternative methods such as nature walks or mindful listening to music can provide the same benefits. Encouraging patients and their families to explore different forms of meditation can empower them to find what resonates best, fostering a sense of agency in their care journey.

Incorporating mindfulness into daily activities can also be beneficial. Mindful eating, for instance, encourages individuals to savor their meals, promoting awareness of hunger cues and food choices, which is particularly important for patients managing vascular health.

Engaging fully in the act of eating can enhance nutrition and overall well-being, while also serving as a moment of calm amid a hectic day. Families can share meals together mindfully, turning mealtime into an opportunity for connection and emotional support, which is crucial during times of stress.

Finally, support groups can serve as an essential resource for families navigating the complexities of vascular dementia. These groups often incorporate mindfulness practices, providing a space to share experiences while learning stress reduction techniques. Connecting with others facing similar challenges can alleviate feelings of isolation and foster a sense of community. By integrating mindfulness and stress reduction into their lives, both patients and their families can cultivate greater emotional well-being, enhancing their overall quality of life while navigating the journey of vascular dementia.

Chapter 5: Caregiver Support Strategies

Understanding the Caregiver Role

The caregiver role in the context of vascular dementia is multifaceted and can be both rewarding and challenging. Caregivers often find themselves navigating a complex landscape of emotional, physical, and cognitive demands as they support their loved ones. Understanding the nuances of this role is crucial for both caregivers and the families of those affected by vascular dementia. Caregivers provide not only practical assistance with daily activities but also emotional support, helping to maintain dignity and quality of life for individuals living with this condition.

One of the primary responsibilities of caregivers is to monitor and assist with daily living activities that may become increasingly difficult for patients with vascular dementia. These activities include personal hygiene, meal preparation, and medication management. Caregivers must be attuned to the changing needs of their loved ones, adapting their approaches as cognitive and physical abilities fluctuate. This requires patience, empathy, and a willingness to learn about the specific challenges associated with vascular dementia. By understanding these challenges, caregivers can foster a supportive environment that prioritizes the health and well-being of the patient.

Communication is another critical aspect of the caregiver role, as individuals with vascular dementia may experience changes in language and comprehension. Caregivers must learn effective communication strategies that promote understanding and reduce frustration. This may involve using simple language, maintaining eye contact, and allowing ample time for responses. Additionally, caregivers often need to advocate for their loved ones, ensuring that their needs are met within healthcare settings. Developing strong communication skills is essential for navigating the complexities of care and fostering a sense of connection.

The emotional toll of caregiving can also be significant. Many caregivers experience feelings of isolation, stress, and burnout, making it essential for them to seek support. Accessing community resources and support networks can provide caregivers with the necessary tools to manage their responsibilities and maintain their own well-being. Engaging with others who share similar experiences can foster a sense of belonging and offer practical advice on coping strategies. Recognizing the importance of self-care is vital, as a caregiver's health directly impacts the quality of care they can provide.

Finally, ongoing education about vascular dementia and its progression is an integral part of the caregiver role. Understanding the condition can empower caregivers to make informed decisions regarding treatment options, lifestyle interventions, and rehabilitation techniques. Staying updated on research advances and emerging therapies can provide hope and direction in the caregiving journey. As caregivers become more knowledgeable, they can better support their loved ones in navigating the challenges of vascular dementia, ultimately enhancing the quality of life for both the caregiver and the patient.

Coping Mechanisms for Caregivers

Caring for a loved one with vascular dementia can be both rewarding and challenging, often placing significant emotional and physical demands on caregivers. It is essential for caregivers to develop coping mechanisms that promote their well-being while effectively supporting their family members. Recognizing the unique challenges posed by vascular dementia, caregivers can benefit from a range of strategies designed to alleviate stress, enhance resilience, and foster a supportive environment for both themselves and their loved ones.

One effective coping mechanism is establishing a structured routine. Individuals with vascular dementia often thrive on predictability, which can help reduce confusion and anxiety. Caregivers can create daily schedules that include regular meal times, activities, and rest periods. This not only provides stability for the patient but also allows caregivers to allocate time for their own self-care, ensuring they maintain their physical and mental health. Flexibility within this routine can also allow caregivers to adapt to the patient's changing needs while still prioritizing their own well-being.

Support networks play a crucial role in the coping strategies of caregivers. Engaging with family members, friends, and community resources can provide emotional support and practical assistance. Caregivers should not hesitate to reach out for help, whether it is through informal gatherings or structured support groups specifically for those caring for individuals with vascular dementia. Sharing experiences and advice with others facing similar challenges can reduce feelings of isolation and provide valuable insights into effective caregiving practices.

Mindfulness and stress-reduction techniques are essential tools for managing the emotional toll of caregiving. Practices such as meditation, yoga, or even simple breathing exercises can help caregivers cultivate a sense of calm amid the chaos. These activities not only improve mental clarity but also enhance emotional resilience, allowing caregivers to respond more effectively to the challenges of daily caregiving. Incorporating these practices into one's routine can lead to improved overall health and a greater capacity to provide care.

Lastly, caregivers should prioritize their physical health through proper nutrition and exercise. Balanced diets rich in nutrients can bolster energy levels and mental alertness, which are crucial when providing care. Regular physical activity helps alleviate stress and promotes overall well-being. Caregivers might consider joining exercise classes or engaging in outdoor activities, which can also serve as opportunities for socialization. By taking care of their own health, caregivers enhance their ability to support their loved ones, creating a more balanced and fulfilling caregiving experience.

Building a Support Network

Building a support network is crucial for families and patients navigating the complexities of vascular dementia. This condition often brings significant emotional, physical, and logistical challenges, making it essential to establish connections with individuals and groups that can provide assistance. A support network typically includes family members, friends, healthcare professionals, and community resources, all of which play a vital role in fostering an environment conducive to managing the disease effectively. By building a robust support system, families can better address the needs of their loved ones while also ensuring their own well-being.

Family members often serve as the first line of support, but they may require additional resources to navigate the complexities of vascular dementia. Open communication among family members is fundamental to creating a supportive atmosphere. Regular family meetings can help everyone stay informed about the patient's condition and care needs. Engaging in these discussions allows family members to express their concerns, share experiences, and collaborate on strategies to improve the quality of life for the person affected. It is also important for families to educate themselves about vascular dementia, which can empower them to make informed decisions regarding care and treatment options.

Healthcare professionals, including doctors, nurses, and social workers, are invaluable assets in the support network. They can provide insights into the latest research, treatment options, and rehabilitation techniques tailored to vascular dementia. Establishing a relationship with a primary care physician who understands the nuances of the condition can facilitate early detection and timely interventions. Additionally, mental health professionals can offer counseling services to both patients and caregivers, helping them cope with the emotional stress that often accompanies the disease. Accessing professional guidance can alleviate feelings of isolation and uncertainty.

Community resources also play a significant role in building a support network. Local organizations often offer support groups, workshops, and educational programs specifically designed for families affected by vascular dementia. These resources provide opportunities for individuals to connect with others facing similar challenges, fostering a sense of camaraderie and shared understanding. Many communities also have respite care services, which can give caregivers a much-needed break while ensuring that their loved ones receive quality care. Utilizing these resources can enhance the overall support system and improve the well-being of both patients and caregivers.

Lastly, it is essential to recognize the importance of self-care for caregivers within the support network. Caring for someone with vascular dementia can be overwhelming, making it imperative for caregivers to seek support for their own mental and physical health. Engaging in support groups or therapy can help caregivers process their experiences and emotions. Moreover, maintaining a healthy lifestyle through proper nutrition, exercise, and social activities can significantly impact their ability to provide care. A well-rounded support network not only aids the person with vascular dementia but also nurtures the caregivers, ensuring that everyone involved can navigate this journey with resilience and strength.

Chapter 6: Medications and Pharmacological Treatments

Overview of Current Medications

In the management of vascular dementia, understanding the landscape of current medications is crucial for families and patients. While there is no cure for vascular dementia, certain medications can help manage symptoms and improve quality of life. These medications can be categorized into several classes, including cholinesterase inhibitors, memantine, and medications targeting vascular health. Each category serves a distinct purpose, and awareness of these options can empower families in discussions with healthcare providers.

Cholinesterase inhibitors, such as donepezil, rivastigmine, and galantamine, are commonly prescribed to enhance cognitive function. These medications work by increasing the levels of acetylcholine, a neurotransmitter involved in memory and learning. While research indicates that these medications may offer modest benefits in some patients with vascular dementia, their effectiveness can vary. It is essential for families to monitor any changes in symptoms and report these to healthcare providers, as individual responses can differ significantly.

Memantine is another medication that may be beneficial, particularly for patients with moderate to severe vascular dementia. This drug works by regulating glutamate, a neurotransmitter that plays a role in learning and memory. Memantine has been shown to help with cognitive symptoms and may also improve daily functioning. Families should discuss the potential for this medication with their healthcare team, especially if cognitive decline appears more pronounced.

In addition to medications directly targeting cognitive symptoms, managing vascular health is critical. Medications that control blood pressure, cholesterol, and diabetes can significantly impact the progression of vascular dementia. By addressing underlying vascular conditions, families can potentially slow the progression of dementia. Healthcare providers often emphasize the importance of a comprehensive approach that includes lifestyle interventions, such as dietary changes and physical activity, in conjunction with pharmacological treatments.

It is vital for families to engage in open dialogues with healthcare professionals regarding the benefits and side effects of medications. This communication can lead to informed decisions that align with the patient's needs and preferences. Regular follow-ups are essential to assess the effectiveness of medications and make necessary adjustments. Ultimately, a thorough understanding of current medications can help families navigate the complexities of vascular dementia, ensuring that their loved ones receive the best possible care and support.

Potential Side Effects and Management

Vascular dementia, like any medical condition, can present a range of potential side effects, particularly related to the cognitive and physical challenges it imposes on patients. Cognitive impairments may manifest as memory loss, difficulty concentrating, or changes in personality. These symptoms can vary in severity and can significantly impact daily living activities. Patients may also experience emotional distress, including anxiety and depression, which can be exacerbated by the loss of independence and the challenges of adapting to cognitive changes. It is crucial for families to recognize these potential side effects early, as timely management can improve the quality of life for both patients and caregivers.

Management of the cognitive and emotional side effects associated with vascular dementia often involves a multifaceted approach. Cognitive rehabilitation techniques, such as memory training and problem-solving exercises, can help patients maintain cognitive functions for as long as possible. Engaging in structured activities that stimulate the mind, such as puzzles or memory games, can also be beneficial. Additionally, emotional support through counseling or support groups can provide a safe space for patients and families to express their feelings and share experiences. Encouraging open communication about the challenges faced can foster a supportive environment that aids in coping.

Nutrition and lifestyle interventions play a vital role in managing the side effects of vascular dementia. A heart-healthy diet rich in fruits, vegetables, whole grains, and omega-3 fatty acids has been associated with improved vascular health, which may help mitigate some cognitive decline. Regular physical activity is equally important, as it not only promotes cardiovascular health but also enhances mood and cognitive function. Families can work together to create a balanced meal plan and encourage participation in physical activities, making lifestyle changes a collective effort that strengthens bonds and improves overall well-being.

Pharmacological treatments also have a place in managing the symptoms of vascular dementia. While there is no cure, certain medications can help alleviate specific symptoms or slow the progression of cognitive decline. It is essential for families to engage in discussions with healthcare providers about the potential benefits and risks associated with these medications. Monitoring for side effects, such as dizziness, fatigue, or gastrointestinal issues, is crucial for ensuring that the treatment remains effective and tolerable. Careful management of medications can help maintain the patient's quality of life while addressing the cognitive and emotional challenges of vascular dementia.

Finally, caregivers play an instrumental role in managing the potential side effects of vascular dementia. Support strategies for caregivers can include respite care, educational resources, and community support networks. Understanding the condition, its progression, and available resources can empower caregivers to provide better care and maintain their own well-being. By recognizing the signs of stress and seeking assistance when needed, caregivers can help ensure that both they and their loved ones navigate the journey of vascular dementia with resilience and support.

Future Directions in Pharmacological Research

Future directions in pharmacological research for vascular dementia are focused on developing targeted therapies that address the underlying vascular issues contributing to cognitive decline. Current medications primarily aim to alleviate symptoms rather than tackle the root causes of vascular dementia. Researchers are now exploring novel compounds that can improve blood flow to the brain, enhance neuroprotection, and promote neurogenesis. This shift towards a more comprehensive approach holds promise for not only improving quality of life for patients but also potentially slowing the progression of the disease.

Another promising avenue of research is the investigation of existing medications that may have applications in vascular dementia treatment. Some studies are examining the effects of antihypertensive drugs or statins, traditionally used for cardiovascular issues, on cognitive function in patients with vascular dementia. Early findings suggest that these medications may have neuroprotective properties that could help mitigate cognitive decline. Such repurposing of drugs could expedite the availability of effective treatments, offering hope to families navigating this challenging condition.

In addition to pharmacological developments, there is a growing interest in the integration of lifestyle interventions with medication regimens. Research indicates that a combination of pharmacological treatments and lifestyle modifications—such as diet, exercise, and cognitive training—can enhance therapeutic outcomes. Future studies are likely to focus on how these combined approaches can be tailored to individual patient needs, thereby maximizing their effectiveness. This holistic view emphasizes the importance of treating vascular dementia through multifaceted strategies that address both biological and lifestyle factors.

Ethical considerations in the development and implementation of new treatments also play a crucial role in future pharmacological research. As new therapies emerge, it is essential to ensure that they are accessible and affordable for patients and their families. Furthermore, clinical trials must prioritize patient safety and informed consent, especially given the vulnerability of individuals with cognitive impairments. Engaging families in the research process can provide valuable insights into patient needs and preferences, fostering a more patient-centered approach to drug development.

Lastly, collaboration between researchers, healthcare providers, and community support networks will be vital in advancing pharmacological research. By fostering partnerships that include caregivers and patients, the research community can gain a deeper understanding of the daily challenges faced by those living with vascular dementia. These insights can guide the focus of future studies and help bridge the gap between laboratory findings and real-world applications, ultimately enhancing care and support for families affected by this condition.

Chapter 7: The Role of Vascular Health

Connection Between Vascular Health and Dementia

The connection between vascular health and dementia is increasingly recognized as crucial in understanding the onset and progression of vascular dementia. Vascular dementia primarily results from impaired blood flow to the brain, often due to conditions that affect blood vessels, such as hypertension, diabetes, and high cholesterol. When these conditions are not managed effectively, they can lead to the deterioration of cognitive functions. This relationship emphasizes the importance of maintaining vascular health as a preventive strategy against dementia. Family members and caregivers play a vital role in monitoring these health parameters and facilitating medical interventions when necessary.

Research indicates that poor vascular health can contribute to cognitive decline in various ways. Reduced blood flow can lead to brain cell damage and death, resulting in memory loss and difficulty with reasoning or problem-solving. Additionally, vascular conditions can cause small strokes or transient ischemic attacks, which can further exacerbate cognitive impairment. Understanding these mechanisms can help families recognize the signs of vascular dementia early, allowing for timely medical evaluation and intervention. This awareness is essential for both patients and their loved ones in navigating the complexities of the condition.

The lifestyle choices and nutritional habits of individuals significantly influence vascular health and, by extension, cognitive function. Diets high in saturated fats and sugars can increase the risk of vascular diseases, while a balanced diet rich in fruits, vegetables, and whole grains can promote better vascular health. Regular physical activity, smoking cessation, and maintaining a healthy weight are also vital in reducing the risk of conditions that lead to vascular dementia. Families can support patients by encouraging healthy lifestyle changes and by participating in activities that promote both physical and mental well-being.

Caregiver support strategies are integral to managing the connection between vascular health and dementia. Education on the importance of regular health check-ups, medication adherence, and lifestyle modifications can empower caregivers to take a proactive role in the patient's health journey. Furthermore, caregivers should be aware of the potential emotional and physical stress associated with managing a loved one's vascular health and dementia symptoms. Connecting with community resources, support groups, and healthcare professionals can provide essential guidance and relief for caregivers, enhancing their ability to support the patient effectively.

As research advances, new insights into the connection between vascular health and dementia continue to emerge. Ongoing studies are exploring how interventions aimed at improving vascular health can potentially slow the progression of cognitive decline. These findings highlight the importance of early detection and diagnosis of vascular dementia, as well as the need for comprehensive care strategies that encompass both medical and lifestyle interventions. Families should remain informed about these developments, as they can significantly impact the management and quality of life for individuals living with vascular dementia.

Preventive Measures for Vascular Health

Preventive measures for vascular health play a crucial role in reducing the risk of vascular dementia and enhancing overall cognitive function. Maintaining optimal vascular health involves a combination of lifestyle choices, dietary adjustments, and regular health screenings. It is essential for families and patients to understand that proactive management of cardiovascular health can significantly impact the likelihood of developing vascular dementia. This knowledge empowers families to take actionable steps that can lead to better outcomes in cognitive health.

One of the key preventive strategies is to adopt a heart-healthy diet. The Mediterranean diet, rich in fruits, vegetables, whole grains, lean proteins, and healthy fats, has been shown to support vascular health.

Families should prioritize foods high in antioxidants and omega-3 fatty acids, such as fatty fish, nuts, and seeds, while limiting saturated fats, trans fats, and added sugars. Educating patients about nutritional choices can foster healthier eating habits, contributing to improved circulation and brain health. Regularly incorporating these dietary principles can also help manage existing health conditions, such as hypertension and diabetes, which are significant risk factors for vascular dementia.

Physical activity is another essential component of preventive measures. Engaging in regular exercise can enhance cardiovascular fitness and promote better blood flow, which is vital for brain health. Families are encouraged to find enjoyable physical activities that can be done together, whether it's walking, swimming, or dancing. Aim for at least 150 minutes of moderate aerobic activity each week, as this can help lower blood pressure, strengthen the heart, and reduce the risk of cognitive decline. Encouraging patients to remain active not only supports vascular health but also enhances mood and overall well-being.

Monitoring and managing blood pressure, cholesterol levels, and blood sugar is critical in preventing vascular dementia. Regular health check-ups allow for early detection and intervention of cardiovascular issues. Families should be proactive in discussing these health metrics with healthcare providers and understanding the importance of medication adherence when prescribed. Implementing regular screenings and following personalized care plans can help mitigate risks associated with vascular health, thus reducing the chance of developing dementia-related complications.

Lastly, stress management and cognitive engagement are vital preventive measures. Chronic stress can negatively impact vascular health and cognitive function, so it is important to adopt stress-reducing practices such as mindfulness, meditation, or yoga. Encouraging patients to engage in mentally stimulating activities—such as puzzles, reading, or social interactions—can help build cognitive resilience. Caregivers should also seek support from community resources and networks that provide information and assistance in managing both their own well-being and that of the patient. By fostering a supportive environment, families can enhance the quality of life for those at risk of vascular dementia while promoting better vascular health for all.

Monitoring and Maintaining Vascular Health

Monitoring and maintaining vascular health is crucial for individuals at risk of or living with vascular dementia. Vascular dementia is often linked to conditions that affect blood flow to the brain, such as hypertension, diabetes, and high cholesterol. Regular monitoring of these risk factors is essential for early detection and management. Family members and caregivers should be aware of their loved ones' health metrics, including blood pressure readings, glucose levels, and lipid profiles. Keeping track of these measurements can help identify any concerning trends that may warrant medical attention and intervention.

In addition to tracking vital signs, adopting a proactive approach to lifestyle modifications can significantly impact vascular health. Encouraging a balanced diet rich in fruits, vegetables, whole grains, and lean proteins can help manage cholesterol and blood sugar levels. Furthermore, regular physical activity plays a vital role in maintaining cardiovascular health. Families can support loved ones by engaging them in physical activities tailored to their abilities, whether it's walking, swimming, or participating in light aerobic exercises. These interventions contribute not only to physical well-being but also to cognitive health, potentially slowing the progression of vascular dementia.

Medication management is another critical aspect of maintaining vascular health. Many individuals with vascular dementia may require medications to control underlying conditions such as hypertension or hyperlipidemia. It is essential for families and caregivers to be involved in medication management, ensuring that prescriptions are filled, dosages are taken correctly, and any side effects are monitored. This involvement can foster a sense of security for both the patient and their caregivers and can lead to more effective management of vascular health.

Regular check-ups with healthcare providers are vital for monitoring vascular health and addressing any concerns promptly. During these visits, families should discuss any changes in their loved one's condition, including cognitive or physical changes that may indicate a decline in vascular health. Healthcare providers can offer tailored recommendations for further testing, adjustments in treatment plans, or referrals to specialists. This collaborative approach can empower families to play an active role in their loved one's care and ensure that their vascular health remains a priority.

Community resources and support networks can also be invaluable in maintaining vascular health. Many organizations offer educational resources, support groups, and workshops focused on lifestyle interventions and caregiver strategies. By connecting with these resources, families can gain knowledge and support that enhances their ability to monitor and maintain their loved one's vascular health. Engaging with local healthcare providers, nutritionists, and exercise specialists can create a comprehensive support system that addresses both physical and cognitive needs, ultimately contributing to better outcomes for individuals living with vascular dementia.

Chapter 8: Research Advances in Vascular Dementia

Current Research Trends

Current research trends in vascular dementia are focused on improving early detection methods, understanding the underlying mechanisms of the disease, and exploring innovative treatment options. One significant area of investigation is the identification of biomarkers that can indicate the presence of vascular dementia before clinical symptoms manifest. Researchers are examining various biological markers in blood and imaging techniques to enhance diagnostic accuracy. These advancements aim to facilitate timely interventions, allowing families to implement care strategies sooner and potentially slow the progression of cognitive decline.

Another critical trend involves the exploration of cognitive rehabilitation techniques tailored for individuals with vascular dementia. Studies are increasingly highlighting the effectiveness of personalized cognitive training programs that take into account each patient's unique cognitive profile. Such interventions not only aim to improve cognitive function but also focus on enhancing the quality of life for patients. Family involvement in these rehabilitation efforts is also being emphasized, as supportive environments can significantly bolster the effectiveness of cognitive therapies.

Nutrition and lifestyle interventions are gaining traction as vital components in managing vascular dementia. Current research is investigating the impact of diet on vascular health and cognitive function, with particular attention paid to the Mediterranean diet and its potential benefits. Studies indicate that diets rich in fruits, vegetables, whole grains, and healthy fats may help mitigate the risk factors associated with vascular dementia. Alongside dietary changes, researchers are also looking into the role of physical activity and social engagement in maintaining cognitive health, suggesting that a holistic approach is essential for optimal outcomes.

In the realm of pharmacological treatments, ongoing studies are assessing the efficacy of various medications aimed at alleviating symptoms and slowing disease progression. Research is exploring the use of existing medications, such as those for hypertension and cholesterol, as well as novel pharmacological agents that target vascular health directly. The goal is to develop comprehensive treatment plans that combine medication with lifestyle modifications, providing a multifaceted approach to managing vascular dementia.

Finally, caregiver support strategies are increasingly recognized as essential in the research landscape. Studies are examining the psychological and emotional impact of caregiving on families and identifying effective support mechanisms. Innovative programs aimed at educating caregivers about vascular dementia, stress management techniques, and community resources are being developed. These efforts not only empower caregivers but also promote a better understanding of the disease within the family unit, fostering a more supportive environment for those living with vascular dementia.

Emerging Therapies and Treatments

Emerging therapies and treatments for vascular dementia are continually evolving, driven by ongoing research and a deeper understanding of the disease's mechanisms. Current approaches focus on modifying risk factors, enhancing cognitive function, and improving the quality of life for patients. While traditional pharmacological treatments have been the mainstay, there is a growing interest in non-pharmacological interventions that address both physical health and cognitive rehabilitation. This shift reflects a holistic approach to managing vascular dementia, encompassing medical, psychological, and lifestyle factors.

One promising area of research involves cognitive rehabilitation techniques tailored specifically for individuals with vascular dementia. These techniques aim to improve cognitive functioning through structured activities that engage memory, attention, and problem-solving skills. Family involvement in these activities can be crucial, as it not only provides support but also fosters a sense of connection and purpose for the patient. Engaging in cognitive exercises, such as memory games or puzzles, can lead to noticeable improvements in daily functioning and overall well-being.

In addition to cognitive rehabilitation, nutrition and lifestyle interventions have garnered attention for their potential benefits in managing vascular dementia. Diets rich in fruits, vegetables, whole grains, and healthy fats, such as the Mediterranean diet, have been associated with better brain health. Regular physical activity and maintaining cardiovascular health through activities like walking or swimming are equally important, as they can enhance blood flow to the brain and reduce the risk of further cognitive decline. These lifestyle changes can empower patients and their families to take an active role in managing the condition.

Pharmacological treatments remain a critical component of managing vascular dementia, although the focus is shifting toward personalized medicine. Research is exploring various medications that target specific symptoms and underlying vascular issues. Additionally, emerging therapies, such as the use of neuroprotective agents, are being studied for their potential to mitigate cognitive decline. Families should work closely with healthcare providers to understand the latest options available and participate in shared decision-making regarding treatment plans.

As advancements in research continue to unfold, the role of community resources and support networks becomes increasingly vital for families navigating vascular dementia. Support groups, educational workshops, and caregiver training programs can provide invaluable assistance, helping families cope with the challenges of the disease. These resources not only offer emotional and practical support but also foster connections among families facing similar experiences. Staying informed and engaged with these emerging therapies and treatments can empower families to advocate for the best possible care for their loved ones.

Future Directions in Vascular Dementia Research

As our understanding of vascular dementia evolves, researchers are increasingly focused on identifying early biomarkers that can facilitate timely diagnosis. Advances in neuroimaging techniques, such as MRI and PET scans, are showing promise in detecting subtle changes in brain structure and function associated with vascular dementia. These innovations may lead to non-invasive methods to identify individuals at risk before significant cognitive decline occurs. Families should stay informed about these developments, as they may soon provide critical insights for early intervention and management.

Another significant area of research is the exploration of cognitive rehabilitation techniques tailored specifically for vascular dementia patients. Studies are investigating the effectiveness of various therapies, including cognitive training, memory exercises, and engagement in social activities. The goal is to enhance cognitive function and improve quality of life. Families can play a crucial role in supporting these interventions by encouraging participation and creating a stimulating environment that fosters cognitive engagement.

Nutrition and lifestyle interventions are also gaining attention as potential preventive measures against vascular dementia. Researchers are examining the impact of diet, physical activity, and lifestyle choices on brain health. Evidence suggests that diets rich in fruits, vegetables, whole grains, and healthy fats may contribute to better vascular health and cognitive function. Families can adopt these dietary changes collectively, creating a supportive atmosphere that promotes healthy habits for both patients and caregivers.

Pharmacological treatments for vascular dementia continue to evolve, with ongoing clinical trials assessing the efficacy of various medications. These studies aim to determine the best approaches for managing symptoms and slowing disease progression. Families should be proactive in discussing medication options with healthcare providers and staying updated on new treatment possibilities. Understanding the risks and benefits of these medications can empower families to make informed decisions regarding their loved one's care.

Finally, ethical considerations in managing vascular dementia will remain a critical focus of research. Issues surrounding autonomy, decision-making capacity, and caregiver responsibilities are increasingly under scrutiny. Researchers are exploring how to balance patient dignity with the need for support and intervention. Families should engage in discussions about these ethical dilemmas, fostering a collaborative approach that respects the wishes and needs of the individual living with vascular dementia. By participating in these conversations, families can help shape future research directions that prioritize the well-being of patients and their caregivers.

Chapter 9: Impact on Daily Living Activities

Challenges Faced by Patients

Patients diagnosed with vascular dementia encounter a myriad of challenges that can significantly impact their quality of life and daily functioning. One of the most immediate obstacles is the cognitive decline that often accompanies the condition. Individuals may experience difficulties with memory, problem-solving, and decision-making, which can complicate even routine tasks. This cognitive impairment can lead to frustration and confusion, making it essential for both patients and their families to understand these challenges and approach them with patience and support.

Emotional and psychological challenges also play a critical role in the experience of vascular dementia. Patients often grapple with feelings of loss, anxiety, and depression as they confront their diagnosis and the changes it brings. The awareness of cognitive decline can lead to a profound sense of grief over lost abilities and independence. Families may notice mood swings or withdrawal from social interactions, which can further exacerbate the isolation that many patients feel. Addressing these emotional aspects is vital, as they can significantly affect the patient's overall well-being and willingness to engage in treatment and rehabilitation efforts.

Another significant challenge faced by patients is the management of comorbid conditions, which are common among those with vascular dementia. Many patients have underlying health issues, such as hypertension, diabetes, or heart disease, that require careful management. The interplay between these conditions and vascular dementia can complicate treatment plans and necessitate frequent medical appointments. Families must navigate these complexities while ensuring that their loved ones receive comprehensive care that addresses both cognitive and physical health needs.

Communication barriers can also pose serious challenges for patients and their families. As cognitive abilities decline, patients may struggle to express their thoughts and feelings, leading to misunderstandings and frustration on both sides. Families may find it increasingly difficult to engage in meaningful conversations, which can affect the emotional connection between the patient and their loved ones. Developing effective communication strategies, such as using simple language and providing visual aids, can help bridge this gap and foster a more supportive environment.

Finally, the challenge of accessing appropriate resources and support cannot be overlooked. Patients and their families often face difficulties in finding specialized care, rehabilitation services, and community support networks tailored to those affected by vascular dementia. The landscape of available resources can be overwhelming, and families may not know where to turn for help. It is crucial for families to seek out educational materials, community organizations, and healthcare providers who understand vascular dementia and can guide them through the complexities of managing the condition. By addressing these challenges collectively, patients and families can better navigate the journey of vascular dementia and enhance their overall quality of life.

Strategies for Daily Living Support

Daily living support for individuals with vascular dementia is crucial in maintaining their quality of life and ensuring safety. Strategies should be tailored to the unique needs of each person, as the progression of vascular dementia can vary widely. Simple modifications in the living environment can significantly enhance independence and reduce anxiety. For instance, utilizing clear labeling for rooms and essential items can help individuals navigate their surroundings more easily. Additionally, decluttering spaces can minimize distractions and the risk of falls, creating a safer and more manageable environment.

Establishing a consistent daily routine can also provide structure and predictability, which benefits both those living with vascular dementia and their caregivers. Routines can help reduce confusion and anxiety, making it easier for individuals to engage in daily tasks. Incorporating familiar activities, such as gardening or cooking, can serve as valuable cognitive exercises while promoting a sense of achievement. Caregivers should encourage participation in these activities, adapting them to the person's abilities, thus fostering a sense of purpose and connection.

Nutrition plays a significant role in supporting cognitive function and overall well-being in individuals with vascular dementia. A balanced diet rich in fruits, vegetables, whole grains, and lean proteins can help manage vascular health. Caregivers should be informed about the importance of meals that are not only nutritious but also enjoyable for the individual. Meal preparation can be a shared activity, allowing caregivers to engage the person in the process, which can improve appetite and create opportunities for social interaction.

Social engagement is another vital aspect of daily living support for individuals with vascular dementia. Maintaining connections with friends, family, and community resources can significantly enhance emotional well-being. Regular visits from family members or participation in community programs can reduce feelings of isolation. Caregivers should seek out local support groups or activities specifically designed for individuals with dementia, as these can provide both social interaction and cognitive stimulation.

Finally, caregivers themselves require support and resources to manage the challenges of daily living with a loved one affected by vascular dementia. Accessing community resources, such as respite care, training sessions, and informational workshops, can empower caregivers with knowledge and strategies to enhance their caregiving experience. It is essential for caregivers to prioritize their own well-being, as their health directly impacts the quality of care provided. By fostering a supportive environment and utilizing available resources, families can navigate the complexities of daily living support for individuals with vascular dementia more effectively.

Adapting the Home Environment

Adapting the home environment is a crucial aspect of managing vascular dementia, enabling patients to maintain independence and safety while providing support. One of the first steps in this process is to evaluate the current living space and identify potential hazards. Common issues include clutter, poor lighting, and uneven surfaces, which can pose risks for those experiencing cognitive decline. Organizing the home to create clear pathways and reducing clutter can help prevent falls and disorientation. Additionally, ensuring that areas are well-lit, especially stairways and hallways, can significantly enhance safety and comfort.

Incorporating visual aids is another effective strategy for adapting the home environment. Simple modifications such as labels on doors, drawers, and rooms can help individuals with vascular dementia orient themselves more easily. Color-coded systems can also be beneficial, as they provide visual cues that assist in memory recall. For instance, using different colors for various rooms or categories of items can support cognitive functioning and make navigation simpler. This approach not only aids in daily routines but also fosters a sense of familiarity within the home.

Fostering a routine within the home environment can further assist individuals living with vascular dementia. Establishing consistent meal times, exercise schedules, and relaxation periods can create a sense of stability that is comforting for patients. Routines help in reducing anxiety and confusion, as they provide a predictable structure to the day. Caregivers should also be encouraged to participate in these routines, reinforcing their role as supportive figures while promoting engagement in daily activities that stimulate cognitive function.

Creating a calming and comfortable atmosphere is vital for reducing agitation and promoting well-being. Soft furnishings, familiar photographs, and personal mementos can help evoke positive memories and provide emotional comfort. Additionally, minimizing loud noises and distractions can create a serene environment conducive to relaxation and cognitive engagement. It is essential for family members to be observant and responsive to the patient's preferences, as each individual may have unique triggers that either soothe or agitate them.

Lastly, ensuring that the home environment accommodates the nutritional and lifestyle needs of the individual is also important. This includes setting up a designated space for meal preparation that encourages healthy eating habits. Stocking the kitchen with nutritious foods and having easy access to fresh fruits and vegetables can support the overall vascular health of the patient. Moreover, engaging in light physical activities within the home, such as stretching or simple exercises, can enhance physical and cognitive health. By taking these steps, families can create a supportive home environment that not only caters to safety and comfort but also promotes the well-being of those living with vascular dementia.

Chapter 10: Ethical Considerations

Decision-Making and Autonomy

Decision-making and autonomy are critical aspects of the experience of individuals living with vascular dementia, as well as for their families and caregivers. As cognitive abilities decline, the capacity for independent decision-making may be affected, leading to challenges in managing daily activities, healthcare choices, and personal preferences. It is essential for families to understand the nuances of these changes and to promote an environment that encourages autonomy while ensuring safety and well-being.

Early recognition of cognitive impairments allows families to engage in conversations about decision-making preferences. It is crucial to discuss and document the individual's wishes regarding healthcare, financial matters, and living arrangements while they still have the capacity to express their opinions clearly. This proactive approach not only respects the autonomy of the person affected but also provides a roadmap for caregivers and family members when difficult decisions arise later in the progression of the disease.

The role of caregivers becomes increasingly significant as vascular dementia progresses. Caregivers often face the challenge of balancing the need to make decisions in the best interest of the person with dementia while respecting their autonomy. It is important for caregivers to involve the individual in discussions about their care and to consider their preferences whenever possible. Encouraging participation in decision-making, even in small matters, can help maintain a sense of agency and dignity for the individual.

Families should also be aware of the ethical considerations surrounding decision-making in vascular dementia. As cognitive decline impacts judgment, the line between supporting autonomy and making necessary interventions can become blurred. Engaging with healthcare professionals, legal advisors, and ethical committees can provide valuable guidance on how to navigate these complex situations. Clear communication among all parties involved is essential to ensure that the individual's best interests are prioritized.

In addition to healthcare decisions, lifestyle choices, such as nutrition and daily routines, can significantly impact the quality of life for individuals with vascular dementia. Families should work together to create supportive environments that empower the individual to make choices about their diet, physical activity, and social interactions. By fostering a collaborative approach to decision-making, families can help individuals maintain a sense of control and enhance their overall well-being, even in the face of cognitive challenges.

Navigating Ethical Dilemmas

Navigating the complexities of vascular dementia often presents families and caregivers with ethical dilemmas that require careful consideration. These dilemmas can arise in various contexts, such as making decisions about treatment options, managing daily care, or addressing the autonomy of the person affected. It is important for families to recognize that ethical decision-making involves balancing respect for the individual's wishes with the need to ensure their safety and well-being. Engaging in open discussions among family members and healthcare professionals can facilitate a better understanding of the values and preferences of the person living with vascular dementia.

One common ethical issue relates to consent and capacity. As vascular dementia progresses, a person's ability to make informed decisions may diminish. Families may find themselves in situations where they need to determine whether their loved one can participate in decisions regarding their care or treatment. It is crucial to involve healthcare professionals who can assess cognitive capacity and provide guidance on respecting the individual's rights while ensuring they receive appropriate care. Documenting preferences when the person is still capable can help guide decisions during later stages of the disease.

Another ethical consideration involves the use of medications and pharmacological treatments. Families often face decisions about whether to initiate or continue certain medications that may alleviate symptoms but also carry potential side effects. In such cases, weighing the benefits against the risks becomes essential. Additionally, the financial implications of treatment options can add another layer of complexity. Families should have candid discussions with doctors about the goals of treatment, considering both the quality of life for the individual and the financial burden on the family.

Caregiver support strategies also bring ethical dilemmas to the forefront. Family members tasked with caregiving may struggle with feelings of guilt or inadequacy, especially if they are unable to meet all the needs of their loved one. It is vital for families to recognize their own limits and seek external support when necessary. Ethical caregiving involves ensuring that caregivers also take care of their own physical and emotional health, which can ultimately enhance their ability to provide care. Community resources, respite care, and support groups can play a significant role in alleviating the burdens faced by caregivers.

Lastly, the impact of vascular dementia on daily living activities necessitates ethical considerations around autonomy and independence. Families may need to make difficult choices about safety versus independence, such as whether to limit driving or manage finances. Respecting the dignity and preferences of the individual while ensuring their safety is a delicate balance. Engaging the person in conversations about their wishes can empower them and preserve their sense of autonomy, even as they navigate the challenges of vascular dementia. In every ethical dilemma faced, families are encouraged to approach decisions thoughtfully and collaboratively, ensuring that the person's values and preferences remain at the forefront of care.

End-of-Life Considerations

End-of-life considerations in the context of vascular dementia are crucial for both patients and their families. As vascular dementia progresses, individuals face a range of challenges that can impact their quality of life and the decisions made regarding their care. Understanding these considerations can help families navigate the emotional and practical complexities involved, ensuring that loved ones receive the appropriate support and dignity throughout their journey.

One of the primary concerns at this stage is the importance of advanced care planning. Families should engage in discussions about the patient's wishes for end-of-life care, including preferences for medical interventions, resuscitation, and hospice options. This process often involves creating advance directives or living wills that articulate the patient's desires regarding life-sustaining treatments. Open communication within the family and with healthcare providers can help clarify these wishes and reduce confusion when difficult decisions arise.

Additionally, palliative care plays a significant role in managing symptoms and enhancing the quality of life for individuals with vascular dementia nearing the end of life. This specialized care focuses on relieving pain and discomfort, while also addressing emotional and psychological needs. Families are encouraged to consider palliative services, which can provide support not only to the patient but also to caregivers, ensuring that they have the resources needed to cope with the emotional toll of caregiving.

Support networks and community resources are vital as families navigate these challenging times. Many organizations offer counseling, support groups, and educational materials specifically tailored for families affected by vascular dementia. Engaging with these resources can provide emotional support and practical advice, helping families to feel less isolated and more empowered in their caregiving roles. It is essential to seek out these community networks to build a support system that can assist during this difficult phase.

Finally, ethical considerations must be forefront in discussions about end-of-life care for vascular dementia patients. Families may encounter dilemmas regarding autonomy, quality of life, and the appropriateness of certain interventions. Ethical frameworks can guide families in making decisions that honor the patient's dignity while also considering their best interests. Consulting with healthcare professionals who specialize in geriatric care can provide valuable insights into ethical decision-making, ensuring that families feel supported in their choices as they navigate the complexities of end-of-life care.

Chapter 11: Community Resources and Support Networks

Identifying Local Resources

Identifying local resources is a crucial step for families navigating the complexities of vascular dementia. Local resources can provide essential support, information, and assistance tailored to the specific needs of patients and their caregivers. These resources can range from healthcare providers and community organizations to support groups and educational programs. By understanding and accessing these local assets, families can enhance their ability to manage the challenges posed by vascular dementia effectively.

Healthcare providers are often the first point of contact for families dealing with vascular dementia. Primary care physicians, neurologists, and geriatric specialists can offer valuable insights into early detection and diagnosis, as well as appropriate management strategies. It is important for families to establish a good relationship with these healthcare professionals, as they can guide them to further resources, recommend cognitive rehabilitation techniques, and prescribe medications that may alleviate some symptoms associated with the condition. Additionally, they can help families navigate the complexities of vascular health, emphasizing the importance of lifestyle interventions that can play a significant role in managing dementia symptoms.

Community organizations, such as local chapters of the Alzheimer's Association or national dementia advocacy groups, often provide a wealth of information and services. These organizations frequently host workshops, seminars, and support groups specifically for families affected by vascular dementia. Participating in these groups can offer emotional support and practical advice from others who share similar experiences. Furthermore, many of these organizations maintain directories of local services, which can include meal delivery programs, transportation assistance, and respite care for caregivers. Engaging with these resources can empower families to create a supportive environment for their loved ones.

Educational programs offered by local universities or hospitals can also enhance understanding of vascular dementia. These programs often focus on early detection, rehabilitation techniques, and nutrition and lifestyle interventions that can positively affect cognitive health. Families attending such workshops can learn about the latest research advances in vascular dementia, as well as practical strategies to incorporate into daily living. This knowledge not only equips families with tools to improve their loved one's quality of life but also fosters a proactive approach to managing the condition.

Finally, it is vital for families to connect with caregiver support networks in their area. These networks can provide a space for caregivers to share their experiences, discuss strategies, and receive emotional support. Many local resources also offer training sessions that teach caregivers how to handle the unique challenges posed by vascular dementia. By leveraging these support systems, families can alleviate some of the burdens associated with caregiving, ensuring that both patients and caregivers receive the guidance and support they need as they navigate this journey together.

Support Groups and Organizations

Support groups and organizations play a pivotal role for families and patients navigating the complexities of vascular dementia. These groups provide a platform for individuals to share their experiences, challenges, and triumphs in a supportive environment. Family members often find solace in connecting with others facing similar circumstances, while patients benefit from the understanding and camaraderie of those who are experiencing similar cognitive changes. Engaging in these groups can help reduce feelings of isolation and anxiety, fostering a sense of community and shared purpose.

Organizations dedicated to vascular dementia offer a wealth of resources that can aid both patients and their families. They often provide educational materials that focus on early detection and diagnosis, equipping family members with the knowledge to recognize symptoms and seek timely medical advice. Many organizations also conduct workshops and seminars that cover various topics, including cognitive rehabilitation techniques, nutrition, and lifestyle interventions tailored to managing vascular dementia. This information can empower families to make informed decisions regarding care and treatment options.

Caregiver support strategies are another essential focus of these groups. Caregiving can be emotionally and physically taxing, and support groups offer a safe space for caregivers to express their feelings and share coping strategies. These forums often lead to the development of friendships and networks that can provide help in practical ways, such as sharing caregiving tips or organizing respite care. Many organizations also offer training programs that equip caregivers with skills to manage daily challenges effectively and enhance the quality of life for both patients and their caregivers.

Additionally, support groups can facilitate access to medications and pharmacological treatments for vascular dementia. Knowledgeable facilitators often work in partnership with healthcare providers to discuss the latest research advances and treatment options. This collaboration can help families stay informed about new therapies, potential side effects, and medication management strategies, ensuring that they can advocate effectively for their loved ones' needs. Awareness of the role of vascular health in preventing dementia is also emphasized, underscoring the importance of lifestyle modifications.

Finally, the impact of vascular dementia on daily living activities can be overwhelming for families. Support groups and organizations offer practical solutions and resources to help families adapt to the challenges posed by the disease. From assistive technologies to community resources, these organizations serve as a bridge to connecting families with the help they need. By fostering a network of support, they enable families to navigate the journey of vascular dementia with greater resilience, ultimately enhancing the lives of both patients and caregivers.

Utilizing Community Services for Families

Utilizing community services can play a crucial role for families navigating the complexities of vascular dementia. These services offer a range of resources that can help enhance the quality of life for both patients and caregivers. Accessing community support can provide necessary information, emotional support, and practical assistance, which are vital in managing the challenges associated with early detection and diagnosis of vascular dementia. Understanding how to leverage these resources can empower families and foster a supportive environment for those affected.

Local community services often include educational programs aimed at increasing awareness of vascular dementia. These programs can provide families with essential information about the condition, its progression, and effective management strategies. Workshops and seminars led by healthcare professionals can equip families with knowledge about cognitive rehabilitation techniques and lifestyle interventions that may slow the progression of the disease. By participating in these educational opportunities, families can become proactive in their approach, enabling them to make informed decisions about care and treatment.

Caregiver support groups are another valuable community resource. Engaging with others who are experiencing similar challenges can alleviate feelings of isolation and stress. These groups often provide a safe space to share experiences, discuss coping strategies, and exchange practical advice. Additionally, support groups may offer guidance on navigating the healthcare system, understanding medications and pharmacological treatments, and accessing other vital services. Connecting with peers can enhance emotional resilience, which is essential for caregivers managing the day-to-day realities of vascular dementia.

Nutrition and lifestyle interventions are critical components of managing vascular health and can often be supported by community resources. Many local organizations provide nutrition counseling, cooking classes, and wellness programs tailored to individuals with vascular dementia. These services can help families implement dietary changes that promote vascular health, thereby potentially delaying the onset of cognitive decline. Furthermore, community fitness programs designed for older adults can encourage physical activity, which is beneficial for both physical and mental well-being.

Finally, families must remain aware of the various community resources that can support them throughout their journey. Local health departments, non-profit organizations, and even faith-based groups often offer services such as respite care, transportation assistance, and legal resources for planning and decision-making. Identifying and utilizing these resources can significantly ease the burden on families and improve the overall quality of care for those living with vascular dementia. By actively engaging with community services, families can create a network of support that addresses both immediate needs and long-term considerations in managing vascular dementia.